OVARIAN CANCER DIET COOKBOOK

Guide To Managing Cancer Through Nutrition - Delicious Recipes, Meal Plans, And Essential Dietary Strategies To Support Treatment, Boost Immunity, And Enhance Well-Being

STEPHANIE LOUDER

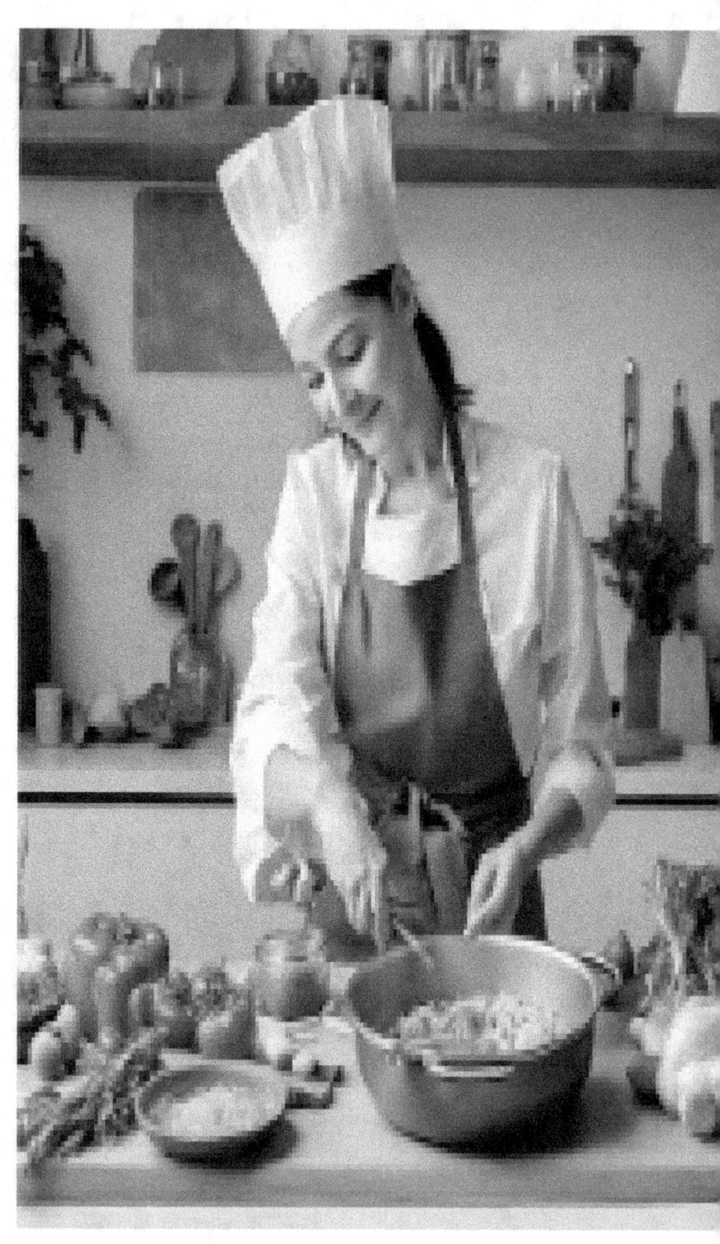

Contents

Disclaimer

This book authored by Stephanie Louder, is provided for informational purposes only.

Neither the author nor the publisher assumes any responsibility for the use or misuse of the information herein. This guide does not endorse or support any specific platform or method. Readers are encouraged to consult with healthcare professionals for personalized advice.

CHAPTER 1
Understanding Ovarian Cancer And Nutrition

Ovarian cancer is a complex and challenging disease that affects thousands of women worldwide each year. Understanding the intricacies of ovarian cancer and its relationship with nutrition is crucial for patients undergoing treatment and recovery. This comprehensive guide delves into the various aspects of ovarian cancer, nutrition, key nutrients, and dietary recommendations to support patients in their journey towards recovery.

Introduction to Ovarian Cancer

Ovarian cancer is a type of cancer that begins in the ovaries, the female reproductive organs responsible for producing eggs and hormones like estrogen and progesterone. It is often referred to as the "silent killer" because symptoms may not manifest until the disease has progressed to advanced stages.

Common symptoms include abdominal bloating, pelvic or abdominal pain, difficulty eating or feeling full quickly, and changes in bowel habits.

There are several types of ovarian cancer, including epithelial ovarian cancer, which arises from the cells on the surface of the ovary, and germ cell tumors, which develop from the cells that produce eggs. The exact cause of ovarian cancer is not fully understood, but factors such as genetics, family history, age, reproductive history, and hormonal factors can contribute to its development.

Diagnosis typically involves imaging tests like ultrasound and CT scans, blood tests to measure tumor markers like CA-125, and biopsy to confirm the presence of cancer cells. Treatment options vary depending on the stage and type of ovarian cancer but often include surgery, chemotherapy, targeted therapy, and radiation therapy.

Nutrition plays a crucial role in the management of ovarian cancer and can significantly impact patients' overall health and well-being during treatment and recovery. A balanced and nutritious diet can help support the immune system, reduce inflammation, manage side effects of treatment, maintain a healthy weight, and improve quality of life.

One of the key goals of nutrition in ovarian cancer recovery is to provide the body with essential nutrients while managing symptoms and treatment-related side effects. This may involve customizing dietary plans based on individual needs, preferences, and treatment protocols. Working closely with healthcare providers, registered dietitians, and nutritionists can help patients develop personalized nutrition plans that optimize their health outcomes.

Key Nutrients for Ovarian Cancer Patients

Several key nutrients play vital roles in supporting ovarian cancer patients' health and recovery.

These nutrients can help boost the immune system, promote healing, manage side effects, and enhance overall well-being. Some of the essential nutrients for ovarian cancer patients include:

1.   Protein: Adequate protein intake is essential for maintaining muscle mass, supporting immune function, and aiding in tissue repair. Good sources of protein include lean meats, poultry, fish, eggs, dairy products, legumes, and plant-based proteins like tofu and tempeh.

2.   Omega-3 Fatty Acids: Omega-3 fatty acids have anti-inflammatory properties and may help reduce inflammation associated with cancer and its treatments. Sources of omega-3 fatty acids include fatty fish like salmon, mackerel, sardines, flaxseeds, chia seeds, walnuts, and soybeans.

3.   Antioxidants: Antioxidants such as vitamins C and E, beta-carotene, and selenium can help protect cells from damage caused by free radicals and oxidative stress.

Fruits, vegetables, nuts, seeds, whole grains, and legumes are rich sources of antioxidants.

4.   Fiber: A diet high in fiber can aid in digestion, promote bowel regularity, and support overall gut health. Foods rich in fiber include whole grains, fruits, vegetables, legumes, nuts, and seeds.

5.   Calcium and Vitamin D: Adequate calcium and vitamin D intake is important for bone health, especially for patients undergoing treatments that may affect bone density. Dairy products, fortified plant-based milk, green leafy vegetables, and sunlight exposure are sources of calcium and vitamin D.

6.   Fluids: Staying hydrated is crucial for patients undergoing cancer treatment to prevent dehydration, support kidney function, and manage side effects like nausea and constipation. Drinking water, herbal teas, and consuming hydrating foods like fruits and vegetables can help maintain hydration levels.

In addition to focusing on key nutrients, ovarian cancer patients should consider specific foods to include and avoid to optimize their nutrition and overall health:

Foods to Include:

1.   Fruits and Vegetables: Colorful fruits and vegetables are rich in vitamins, minerals, antioxidants, and phytochemicals that can support immune function, reduce inflammation, and promote overall health. Aim to include a variety of colors and types of fruits and vegetables in your diet.

2.   Whole Grains: Choose whole grains like brown rice, quinoa, oats, barley, and whole wheat bread and pasta to increase fiber intake and support digestive health.

3.   Lean Protein: Include lean sources of protein such as skinless poultry, fish, tofu, legumes, and nuts to meet your protein needs without excess saturated fat.

4. Healthy Fats: Incorporate sources of healthy fats like avocados, olive oil, nuts, and seeds in moderation to support heart health and overall well-being.

5. Hydrating Foods: Consume hydrating foods like soups, broths, fruits, vegetables, and herbal teas to maintain hydration levels, especially if you experience nausea or difficulty drinking large amounts of fluids.

Foods to Avoid or Limit:

1. Processed Foods: Minimize intake of processed foods high in added sugars, unhealthy fats, and sodium, as they can contribute to inflammation and negatively impact overall health.

2. Sugary Beverages: Limit consumption of sugary drinks like soda, fruit juices, and energy drinks, as they can contribute to weight gain and increase inflammation.

3. High-Fat Foods: Reduce consumption of high-fat foods like fried foods, fatty cuts of meat, full-fat dairy products, and excessive amounts of

added oils, as they can contribute to weight gain and cardiovascular risk.

4.   Alcohol: Limit alcohol intake, as excessive alcohol consumption can increase the risk of certain cancers and negatively impact overall health.

5.   Sodium: Monitor sodium intake and avoid high-sodium foods like processed meats, canned soups, and salty snacks, as they can contribute to fluid retention and high blood pressure.

By incorporating nutrient-dense foods, staying hydrated, and following dietary recommendations tailored to individual needs, ovarian cancer patients can support their recovery, manage treatment-related side effects, and improve their overall quality of life. Working closely with healthcare providers, including oncologists, dietitians, and nutritionists, can help patients develop and maintain healthy eating habits throughout their cancer journey.

CHAPTER 2
Breakfasts For Recovery

Energizing Smoothies And Juices

Energizing smoothies and juices are essential components of a recovery-focused breakfast. These beverages offer a concentrated dose of nutrients in an easily digestible form, making them ideal for individuals who may have limited appetite or need a quick nutrient boost in the morning.

Nutrient Content

Smoothies and juices can be packed with a variety of nutrients, including vitamins, minerals, antioxidants, and essential fatty acids. Ingredients like leafy greens (spinach, kale), fruits (berries, bananas), nuts and seeds (chia seeds, almonds), and plant-based proteins (pea protein, hemp protein) are commonly used to create nutrient-dense beverages. These nutrients play a crucial role in supporting overall health and aiding in the recovery process.

Hydration and Electrolyte Balance

In addition to nutrients, smoothies and juices contribute to hydration, which is vital for recovery. Including hydrating ingredients like coconut water or adding water-rich fruits such as cucumbers or watermelon helps maintain fluid balance and supports electrolyte replenishment, especially important for individuals recovering from illnesses or intensive physical activities.

Digestive Support

Certain ingredients in smoothies and juices, such as probiotic-rich yogurt or kefir, fiber-rich fruits and vegetables, and digestive enzymes from ingredients like ginger or pineapple, can support digestive health. A healthy digestive system is crucial for nutrient absorption and overall well-being, making these beverages beneficial for recovery.

Customization and Adaptation

One of the advantages of energizing smoothies and juices is their versatility.

They can be customized to meet specific dietary needs, taste preferences, and nutritional goals.

For example, individuals focusing on protein intake may add a scoop of protein powder, while those needing extra fiber may include ingredients like flaxseeds or psyllium husk.

Practical Tips

To make energizing smoothies and juices a part of daily breakfast routines, it's helpful to have a variety of recipes on hand. Preparing smoothie packs with pre-measured ingredients or freezing pre-made smoothies in individual portions can save time and streamline breakfast preparation, particularly for busy mornings.

Nutrient-Packed Breakfast Bowls

Nutrient-packed breakfast bowls offer a balanced combination of carbohydrates, proteins, healthy fats, and essential nutrients in a convenient and customizable format. These bowls are versatile and can be tailored to suit different dietary preferences and specific nutritional needs.

Base Ingredients

A nutrient-packed breakfast bowl typically starts with a base ingredient that provides complex carbohydrates and fiber. Common base options include whole grains like oats, quinoa, or brown rice, which are rich in nutrients like B vitamins, iron, and fiber. Alternatively, individuals may opt for smoothie bowl bases made from blended fruits or vegetables for a lighter option.

Protein Sources

Including a source of protein in breakfast bowls is essential for supporting muscle repair and satiety. Protein-rich additions such as Greek yogurt, tofu, nuts and seeds, or lean animal proteins like eggs or poultry can be incorporated into breakfast bowls to provide a balanced nutrient profile.

Healthy Fats

Healthy fats play a crucial role in promoting heart health, hormone balance, and overall well-being. Adding sources of healthy fats like avocados, nut butters, seeds (chia, flaxseed), or drizzling with olive oil or coconut oil can enhance the nutritional value of breakfast bowls and contribute to a satisfying meal.

Colorful and Nutrient-Dense Toppings

Toppings in breakfast bowls not only add flavor and texture but also contribute additional nutrients. Colorful fruits such as berries, citrus fruits, and tropical fruits provide antioxidants, vitamins, and minerals. Nuts and seeds offer omega-3 fatty acids and micronutrients, while dried fruits can add sweetness and fiber.

Functional Additions

To further boost the nutritional benefits of breakfast bowls, functional ingredients like superfood powders (spirulina, maca, acai), adaptogens (ashwagandha, rhodiola), and herbal supplements (turmeric, ginger) can be included. These additions may have specific health-promoting properties, such as immune support, stress reduction, or anti-inflammatory effects.

Incorporating nutrient-packed breakfast bowls into a meal plan can be simplified with batch cooking and strategic ingredient selection. Preparing larger batches of grains, proteins, and toppings ahead of time allows for quick assembly of breakfast bowls throughout the week. Experimenting with different flavor combinations and ingredient pairings keeps breakfasts exciting and satisfying.

Healing Porridges and Oatmeal Varieties

Healing porridges and oatmeal varieties are comforting and nourishing options for breakfast, especially for individuals focusing on recovery. These dishes offer a warm, soothing texture and can be customized with a range of ingredients to enhance their nutritional content and therapeutic benefits.

Whole Grains and Alternative Options

Porridges and oatmeal are traditionally made with oats, but they can also be prepared using other whole grains like quinoa, millet, or buckwheat for variety and additional nutrients. Using whole grains ensures a good source of complex carbohydrates, fiber, and essential vitamins and minerals.

Gut-Friendly Ingredients

Including gut-friendly ingredients in healing porridges and oatmeal varieties can support digestive health, which is crucial for overall well-being and nutrient absorption. Ingredients like ground flaxseeds, chia seeds, probiotic-rich yogurt or kefir, and fermented foods like miso or sauerkraut can promote a healthy gut microbiome.

Anti-Inflammatory Additions

For individuals dealing with inflammation or recovering from inflammatory conditions, incorporating anti-inflammatory ingredients into porridges and oatmeal can be beneficial. Turmeric, ginger, cinnamon, and omega-3-rich foods like walnuts or flaxseed oil have anti-inflammatory properties and can help reduce inflammation in the body.

Balancing blood sugar levels is important, especially for individuals with conditions like diabetes or insulin resistance. Choosing low-glycemic index (GI) ingredients such as steel-cut oats, quinoa, or adding protein and healthy fats (nuts, seeds, nut butters) to oatmeal can help stabilize blood sugar levels and provide sustained energy.

Enhancing the flavor of healing porridges and oatmeal varieties can be done with natural sweeteners like honey, maple syrup, or mashed fruits (bananas, apples). Spices such as cinnamon, nutmeg, cardamom, and vanilla extract add warmth and depth to the dishes. Incorporating citrus zest, dried fruits, or a drizzle of coconut milk or almond milk can also elevate the taste experience.

The texture and consistency of porridges and oatmeal can be adjusted to individual preferences. Cooking oats longer creates a smoother, creamier texture, while using less liquid results in a thicker, heartier consistency. Adding nuts, seeds, or crunchy toppings like granola provides contrast in texture and enhances the overall eating experience.

Incorporating Superfoods

To boost the nutritional content of healing porridges and oatmeal, superfoods can be incorporated. Examples include goji berries, hemp seeds, spirulina, or matcha powder.

These superfoods are rich in antioxidants, vitamins, and minerals, offering additional health benefits to the breakfast meal.

Temperature and Serving Suggestions

Healing porridges and oatmeal varieties can be served hot, warm, or chilled, depending on personal preference and the season. Toppings like fresh fruits, nuts, seeds, and a drizzle of honey or nut butter can be added just before serving to enhance presentation and flavor.

Serving in cozy bowls or mugs adds to the comfort and appeal of these breakfast options.

CHAPTER 3
Wholesome Main Dishes

Creating wholesome main dishes for recovery involves a thoughtful selection of ingredients that prioritize nutrition, flavor, and healing properties. One of the key elements in these dishes is the inclusion of lean protein sources. Lean proteins are essential for recovery as they provide the building blocks for repairing tissues and supporting overall health. Options such as skinless poultry, fish, lean cuts of beef or pork, tofu, tempeh, and legumes like lentils and chickpeas offer a range of nutrients without excess saturated fats or cholesterol.

These proteins can be prepared in various ways, from grilling and baking to sautéing or steaming, allowing for versatility in creating satisfying and nutritious meals.

Incorporating healing grains and legumes further enhances the nutritional profile of main dishes. Whole grains like quinoa, brown rice, barley, and oats are rich in fiber, vitamins, and minerals, promoting digestive health and providing sustained energy. Legumes, including beans, peas, and lentils, are excellent sources of plant-based protein, fiber, and antioxidants.

They contribute to satiety, help regulate blood sugar levels, and support heart health. Combining these grains and legumes with lean proteins creates balanced meals that support recovery by nourishing the body with essential nutrients.

Vegetable-centric main courses are a cornerstone of wholesome dishes for recovery. Vegetables provide a myriad of vitamins, minerals, and phytonutrients that promote overall well-being and aid in the healing process. Incorporating a variety of colorful vegetables ensures a diverse array of nutrients, such as vitamin C, beta-carotene, potassium, and folate. Leafy greens, cruciferous vegetables like broccoli and cauliflower, root vegetables like carrots and sweet potatoes, and vibrant peppers, tomatoes, and onions add both flavor and nutrition to main dishes.

Roasting, stir-frying, or steaming vegetables can preserve their nutrients while enhancing their natural flavors, making them appealing and beneficial additions to recovery-focused meals.

When creating vegetable-centric main courses, it's essential to consider cooking techniques that preserve nutrients and flavors. For example, lightly steaming or stir-frying vegetables can help retain their crispness and vibrant colors while minimizing nutrient loss.

Roasting vegetables with a drizzle of olive oil and herbs adds depth of flavor without excessive calories or unhealthy fats. Incorporating fresh herbs, spices, and citrus juices can further enhance the taste of vegetable-centric dishes, making them satisfying and enjoyable for individuals on a recovery journey.

In summary, wholesome main dishes for recovery encompass a balance of lean protein options, healing grains and legumes, and vegetable-centric courses.

By incorporating these elements into meals, individuals can support their recovery process by nourishing their bodies with essential nutrients, promoting overall health and well-being. Experimenting with different ingredients, cooking techniques, and flavor combinations can result in delicious and nutritious main dishes that contribute to a holistic approach to recovery and wellness.

CHAPTER 4
<u>Brain-Boosting Salads And Dressings</u>

Brain-boosting salads and dressings play a vital role in promoting cognitive health and overall well-being. These dishes are not only delicious but also packed with nutrients that support brain function, memory, and concentration. Incorporating a variety of colorful vegetables, fruits, nuts, seeds, and healthy fats, brain-boosting salads and dressings offer a delightful way to nourish the mind and body.

Salad recipes designed for brain health are characterized by their nutrient density and variety of ingredients. Dark leafy greens like spinach, kale, and arugula are staple components due to their high content of antioxidants, vitamins, and minerals. These greens provide essential nutrients such as vitamin K, which is crucial for brain health and cognitive function. Additionally, including colorful vegetables like bell peppers, tomatoes, carrots, and beets adds a spectrum of vitamins, antioxidants, and fiber, supporting overall brain function and reducing oxidative stress.

Incorporating brain-boosting fruits such as berries, especially blueberries, strawberries, and raspberries, adds a burst of flavor and a wealth of antioxidants, including flavonoids and anthocyanins. These compounds have been linked to improved cognitive function, memory enhancement, and protection against age-related cognitive decline. Nuts and seeds like walnuts, almonds, flaxseeds, and chia seeds are rich in omega-3 fatty acids, essential for brain health and known for their anti-inflammatory properties.

Protein sources like lean chicken, turkey, or plant-based options such as chickpeas, lentils, and tofu can be added to brain-boosting salads to enhance satiety and provide amino acids necessary for neurotransmitter production. Including whole grains like quinoa, brown rice, or farro adds complex carbohydrates for sustained energy and fiber to support gut health, which is closely linked to brain function through the gut-brain axis.

In crafting homemade dressings for brain-boosting salads, using high-quality oils like extra virgin olive oil, avocado oil, or flaxseed oil provides healthy monounsaturated fats and omega-3 fatty acids. These fats are beneficial for brain health, improving cognitive function, and reducing the risk of cognitive decline. Incorporating fresh herbs like basil, parsley, cilantro, or mint adds flavor and additional antioxidants, vitamins, and minerals to the dressing.

Adding citrus juices like lemon, lime, or orange to dressings not only enhances taste but also provides vitamin C, an antioxidant that supports immune function and contributes to brain health. Including ingredients like garlic, ginger, turmeric, and cumin not only adds depth of flavor but also brings anti-inflammatory and neuroprotective properties to the dressing, further enhancing its brain-boosting benefits.

Experimenting with different combinations of ingredients, such as a spinach and berry salad with a citrus vinaigrette or a kale and quinoa salad with a tahini-ginger dressing, offers a diverse range of flavors and nutrients that contribute to optimal brain health. Incorporating these brain-boosting salads and dressings into a balanced diet rich in whole foods, lean proteins, healthy fats, and complex carbohydrates can have significant benefits for cognitive function, memory retention, and overall well-being.

CHAPTER 5
Nourishing Soups And Stews

Nourishing Soups and Stews are foundational elements of a healing and recovery-focused diet. These dishes not only provide warmth and comfort but also deliver essential nutrients that support the body's healing processes. Whether it's a nutrient-rich soup packed with vitamins and minerals or a comforting stew brimming with wholesome ingredients, these culinary creations play a vital role in nourishing the body and promoting overall well-being.

Nutrient-rich soups form a crucial part of a healing diet due to their ability to deliver concentrated doses of essential nutrients in a readily digestible form. These soups are often crafted with a variety of vegetables, herbs, and proteins, creating a harmonious blend of flavors and health benefits. For instance, a vegetable broth-based soup enriched with leafy greens like kale or spinach can provide a wealth of vitamins such as vitamin

A, C, and K, along with minerals like iron and calcium. Additionally, the inclusion of lean proteins such as chicken or tofu adds high-quality protein essential for tissue repair and immune function.

The concept of nutrient-rich soups extends beyond basic broths and encompasses a wide range of culinary styles and cultural influences.

For example, traditional Asian soups like miso soup or Vietnamese pho combine umami-rich ingredients like miso paste or beef broth with nutrient-dense additions like tofu, mushrooms, and fresh herbs, offering a symphony of flavors and health-promoting compounds. Similarly, Mediterranean-inspired soups often feature ingredients like tomatoes, legumes, and olive oil, providing a robust dose of antioxidants, fiber, and heart-healthy fats.

In addition to their nutritional benefits, nutrient-rich soups are also known for their hydrating properties. Soups with a high water content, such as clear broths or vegetable-based soups, contribute to overall hydration levels, which is essential for supporting bodily functions and promoting detoxification. Incorporating hydrating ingredients like cucumbers, celery, and zucchini into soups not only adds moisture but also enhances the overall freshness and vitality of the dish.

Moving on to comforting stews, these hearty dishes are renowned for their ability to provide sustenance and satisfaction during recovery periods. Comforting stews typically feature slow-cooked ingredients such as tender meats, root vegetables, and aromatic spices, resulting in rich flavors and tender textures. One of the key benefits of stews lies in their versatility, allowing for the incorporation of a wide range of nutrient-dense foods tailored to individual dietary needs and preferences.

For individuals undergoing recovery, comforting stews offer a nourishing and easily digestible option that can be customized to meet specific nutritional requirements.

For instance, a beef and vegetable stew can be enriched with nutrient-dense additions like sweet potatoes, carrots, and onions, providing a balanced combination of carbohydrates, proteins, and essential vitamins and minerals. The slow cooking process also helps break down tough cuts of meat, making them more tender and easier to digest, while infusing the broth with depth of flavor and nutrient concentration.

Furthermore, the concept of comforting stews extends beyond meat-based variations to include vegetarian and vegan options that showcase the abundance of plant-based ingredients available for culinary exploration. Lentil stews, for example, are celebrated for their high protein and fiber content, making them a satisfying choice for vegetarians and vegans seeking nourishing meal options.

By incorporating a diverse array of legumes, grains, and vegetables, vegetarian stews offer a nutrient-rich alternative that promotes satiety and supports overall well-being.

Incorporating healing herbs and spices into both soups and stews further enhances their nutritional profile and therapeutic potential. Ingredients like turmeric, ginger, garlic, and fresh herbs not only contribute to the flavor complexity of these dishes but also offer anti-inflammatory, immune-boosting, and digestive benefits.

Turmeric, known for its active compound curcumin, has been studied for its potential to reduce inflammation and support joint health, making it a valuable addition to healing soups and stews, especially for individuals managing inflammatory conditions.

When crafting nourishing soups and stews for healing and recovery, attention to ingredient quality, cooking methods, and flavor balance is paramount. Opting for organic, locally sourced ingredients whenever possible ensures optimal nutrient density and reduces exposure to pesticides and additives.

Utilizing slow cooking techniques such as simmering or braising allows flavors to develop fully while preserving the nutritional integrity of the ingredients. Additionally, mindful seasoning with natural herbs, spices, and healthy fats like olive oil or coconut oil enhances taste without compromising nutritional value.

Nourishing soups and stews represent a cornerstone of a healing-focused diet, offering a delicious and versatile way to deliver essential nutrients, promote hydration, and support overall well-being during recovery periods. Whether enjoying a nutrient-rich vegetable soup or savoring a comforting beef stew, these culinary creations embody the synergy of nourishment and comfort, making them invaluable additions to a holistic approach to health and healing.

CHAPTER 6
Memory-Enhancing Sandwiches And Wraps

Creating memory-enhancing sandwiches and wraps involves combining ingredients that are known to support brain health and cognitive function. These recipes not only provide essential nutrients but also offer convenience for busy days when quick yet nutritious meals are needed.

Let's delve into some ideas for sandwiches and wraps that can boost your brainpower and keep you fueled throughout the day.

Sandwich Ideas with Brain-Boosting Ingredients

When crafting sandwiches for memory enhancement, it's crucial to include ingredients rich in nutrients like omega-3 fatty acids, antioxidants, vitamins, and minerals that support brain function. Here are some sandwich ideas that incorporate these brain-boosting ingredients:

1.   Salmon and Avocado Sandwich: Start with whole-grain bread and layer it with grilled or

smoked salmon, which is abundant in omega-3s. Add slices of creamy avocado for healthy fats, along with leafy greens like spinach or kale for added vitamins and minerals.

2.   Turkey and Spinach Wrap: Use a whole-grain wrap and fill it with lean turkey slices, spinach leaves, and a spread of hummus or mashed avocado. Turkey is a good source of protein, while spinach provides folate and antioxidants crucial for brain health.

3.   Egg and Vegetable Sandwich: Cook scrambled or boiled eggs and place them on whole-grain toast. Add sliced tomatoes, bell peppers, and a sprinkle of feta cheese for a colorful and nutrient-packed sandwich. Eggs offer choline, a nutrient linked to improved memory.

4.   Peanut Butter and Banana Wrap: Spread natural peanut butter on a whole-grain wrap and add sliced bananas. Drizzle with a touch of honey for sweetness.

This combination provides protein, healthy fats, and carbohydrates for sustained energy and brain function.

5.   Chicken and Broccoli Sandwich: Grill or bake chicken breast and place it on whole-grain bread. Add steamed broccoli florets and a spread of Greek yogurt mixed with herbs for a creamy and nutritious sandwich. Broccoli is rich in antioxidants and vitamin K, beneficial for brain health.

6.   Tuna Salad Wrap: Mix canned tuna with Greek yogurt, diced celery, and a squeeze of lemon juice. Spread this mixture on a whole-grain wrap and add lettuce leaves and cucumber slices. Tuna is a source of omega-3s, while vegetables provide additional nutrients and fiber.

7.   Hummus and Veggie Sandwich: Spread hummus on whole-grain bread and layer it with sliced cucumbers, bell peppers, and shredded carrots. Sprinkle with pumpkin or sunflower seeds for added crunch and nutrition.

Hummus offers plant-based protein and fiber, supporting overall brain health.

8. Bean and Avocado Wrap: Mash black beans with mashed avocado and spread it on a whole-grain wrap. Add diced tomatoes, red onion, and cilantro for flavor. Beans are rich in folate and antioxidants, while avocado provides healthy fats and vitamins.

These sandwich ideas showcase a variety of brain-boosting ingredients, including omega-3 fatty acids from fish, antioxidants from colorful vegetables, protein from lean meats and legumes, and healthy fats from avocado and nuts. Incorporating these sandwiches into your diet can contribute to improved cognitive function and overall brain health.

Wrap Recipes for Quick and Nutritious Meals

Wraps are versatile and convenient, making them ideal for busy individuals seeking nutritious meals that can be prepared quickly.

Here are some wrap recipes designed to be both nutritious and time-efficient:

1.   Mediterranean Chicken Wrap: Grill or sauté chicken breast strips with Mediterranean herbs like oregano and thyme. Fill a whole-grain wrap with the cooked chicken, diced tomatoes, cucumbers, olives, and a dollop of tzatziki sauce. This wrap is packed with protein, vegetables, and Mediterranean flavors.

2.   Quinoa and Vegetable Wrap: Cook quinoa according to package instructions and let it cool. Spread hummus on a whole-grain wrap and add cooked quinoa, diced bell peppers, shredded carrots, and baby spinach leaves. Roll it up for a fiber-rich and satisfying meal.

3.   Shrimp and Mango Wrap: Sauté shrimp with a splash of lime juice until cooked. Fill a whole-grain wrap with the shrimp, sliced mango, avocado slices, and a drizzle of mango salsa or a squeeze of lime. This wrap offers a balance of protein, healthy fats, and tropical flavors.

4.   Greek Salad Wrap: Toss diced cucumbers, tomatoes, red onion, Kalamata olives, and feta cheese with a Greek vinaigrette. Spread this salad mixture on a whole-grain wrap and add a few spinach leaves. Roll it up for a refreshing and Mediterranean-inspired wrap.

5.   Spicy Black Bean Wrap: Mash black beans with diced jalapeños, cilantro, and a squeeze of lime juice. Spread this bean mixture on a whole-grain wrap and add shredded lettuce, diced tomatoes, and a sprinkle of grated cheese.

Roll it up and toast it for a warm and flavorful wrap.

6.   Tofu and Vegetable Wrap: Sauté tofu cubes with your favorite spices until golden brown. Fill a whole-grain wrap with the cooked tofu, shredded cabbage, sliced bell peppers, and a drizzle of tahini or peanut sauce. This wrap is a plant-based option rich in protein and fiber.

7.   Caprese Wrap: Layer sliced fresh mozzarella, tomato slices, and basil leaves on a whole-grain wrap.

Drizzle with balsamic glaze or pesto for added flavor.

Roll it up for a classic Italian-inspired wrap that's light yet satisfying.

8.   Smoked Salmon and Cream Cheese Wrap: Spread cream cheese on a whole-grain wrap and add slices of smoked salmon, cucumber ribbons, and dill sprigs. Roll it up and slice it into pinwheels for an elegant and protein-rich snack or meal.

These wrap recipes offer a range of flavors and ingredients while prioritizing nutrition and ease of preparation. Whether you prefer a protein-packed option like the Mediterranean Chicken Wrap or a refreshing choice like the Shrimp and Mango Wrap, incorporating these recipes into your meal rotation can make healthy eating more accessible and enjoyable.

Memory-enhancing sandwiches and wraps can be both delicious and beneficial for brain health.

By choosing ingredients rich in nutrients like omega-3 fatty acids, antioxidants, vitamins, and minerals, you can create meals that support cognitive function and overall well-being. Whether you opt for a salmon and avocado sandwich or a quinoa and vegetable wrap, these recipes offer a convenient way to nourish your body and mind.

CHAPTER 7
Beverages For Brain Boosting

Beverages play a crucial role in our daily lives, not just for quenching thirst but also for nourishing our bodies and enhancing our overall well-being. When it comes to brain health and boosting cognitive function, the choice of beverages becomes even more critical. In this discussion, we'll delve into the realm of beverages specifically designed to boost brain function, with a focus on hydration tips tailored for ovarian cancer patients and brain-enhancing drink recipes that promote cognitive vitality.

Hydration is fundamental to good health, and for individuals undergoing ovarian cancer treatment, maintaining optimal hydration levels is of utmost importance. Chemotherapy and other cancer treatments can often lead to dehydration, making it essential for patients to prioritize hydration as part of their daily routine. Hydration not only helps in flushing out toxins from the body but also supports various bodily functions, including brain function.

One of the key hydration tips for ovarian cancer patients is to ensure a steady intake of fluids throughout the day. This includes not only water but also other hydrating beverages such as herbal teas, coconut water, and clear soups. It's important for patients to monitor their fluid intake and aim for a minimum of eight glasses of fluids per day, adjusting this amount based on their activity levels, climate, and individual hydration needs.

In addition to staying hydrated with fluids, ovarian cancer patients can benefit from incorporating brain-enhancing drink recipes into their daily diet. These recipes are designed to not only provide hydration but also deliver nutrients that support cognitive function and overall brain health.

Let's explore some brain-enhancing drink recipes that can be easily integrated into a patient's meal plan:

1.   Blueberry and Spinach Smoothie: This vibrant smoothie is packed with antioxidants from blueberries and nutrient-rich spinach.

 Antioxidants help protect brain cells from damage and support cognitive function. To make this smoothie, blend together a handful of fresh or frozen blueberries, a handful of spinach leaves, a banana for sweetness, a scoop of Greek yogurt or a plant-based alternative for creaminess, and a splash of almond milk or water. Optionally, add a tablespoon of chia seeds or flaxseeds for an extra boost of omega-3 fatty acids, which are beneficial for brain health.

2.   Turmeric Golden Milk: Turmeric contains curcumin, a compound known for its anti-inflammatory and neuroprotective properties. Golden milk, made with turmeric, is a soothing and nourishing beverage that can be enjoyed warm or cold. To prepare turmeric golden milk, heat a cup of coconut milk or almond milk in a saucepan, add a teaspoon of ground turmeric, a pinch of black pepper (to enhance curcumin

absorption), a dash of cinnamon for flavor, and a natural sweetener like honey or maple syrup to taste. Simmer the mixture for a few minutes, then strain and enjoy.

3.   Green Tea Matcha Latte: Matcha is a powdered form of green tea known for its high antioxidant content and potential cognitive benefits. A green tea matcha latte combines the goodness of matcha with the calming effects of green tea. To make this latte, whisk together a teaspoon of matcha powder with a small amount of hot water to create a smooth paste.

Heat a cup of milk (dairy or plant-based) in a separate saucepan, then pour it over the matcha paste. Sweeten with honey or agave syrup if desired. The combination of caffeine from green tea and the amino acid L-theanine can promote alertness and focus.

4.   Beetroot and Berry Juice: Beetroots are rich in nitrates, which have been linked to

improved blood flow to the brain, potentially enhancing cognitive performance.

Combine beetroot with berries like strawberries, raspberries, or blackberries to create a refreshing and nutrient-packed juice. Simply juice fresh beetroot and berries together, or blend them with a little water and strain for a smoother texture. Add a squeeze of lemon juice for extra flavor and a dash of ginger for a zesty kick.

5.   Omega-3 Rich Smoothie: Omega-3 fatty acids, found abundantly in fatty fish like salmon, are essential for brain health. For those who prefer a plant-based option, flaxseeds, chia seeds, and walnuts are excellent sources of alpha-linolenic acid (ALA), a type of omega-3 fatty acid.

Create an omega-3 rich smoothie by blending together a serving of fatty fish (if using), a tablespoon of ground flaxseeds or chia seeds, a handful of mixed berries, a banana, a scoop of yogurt or a plant-based alternative, and a splash of milk or a milk substitute. This smoothie not only supports brain function but also provides a good balance of nutrients for overall health.

Incorporating these brain-enhancing drink recipes into a well-rounded diet can contribute to improved cognitive function, mental clarity, and overall well-being for ovarian cancer patients and individuals looking to boost their brain health. It's important to consult with a healthcare professional or a registered dietitian to ensure that these beverages align with individual dietary needs and treatment

CHAPTER 8
Quick And Easy Snacks

Quick and easy snacks are a lifesaver for busy days or moments when hunger strikes unexpectedly. These snacks not only satisfy cravings but also provide a quick burst of energy to keep you going. Energy-boosting snack ideas encompass a wide range of options that are not only delicious but also packed with nutrients to fuel your body. When you're on the go, nutritious snacks become essential to maintain a balanced diet and support your active lifestyle.

One of the key aspects of quick and easy snacks is their convenience. These snacks are typically ready to eat or require minimal preparation, making them ideal for hectic schedules. Whether you're at work, school, or traveling, having access to energy-boosting snacks can help you stay focused and energized throughout the day.

When it comes to energy-boosting snack ideas, variety is key.

Incorporating a mix of carbohydrates, protein, and healthy fats can provide a sustained source of energy and prevent energy crashes. For example, a snack like Greek yogurt with berries and a sprinkle of granola combines protein, vitamins, and fiber for a satisfying and nutritious option.

Nutritious snacks for on-the-go are designed to be portable and easy to eat without compromising on health benefits. Options like mixed nuts, fruit slices, whole grain crackers with cheese, or homemade energy bars are great choices that offer a balance of macronutrients and micronutrients. These snacks can be prepped in advance and carried in your bag or lunchbox for whenever hunger strikes.

In addition to providing energy, quick and easy snacks can also contribute to overall health and well-being. Choosing nutrient-dense snacks over processed foods high in sugar and unhealthy fats can support weight management, improve mood and concentration, and enhance physical performance.

When planning energy-boosting snack ideas, consider your individual dietary needs and preferences. Whether you follow a specific diet like vegetarian, vegan, or gluten-free, there are plenty of snack options available to suit your lifestyle. Experimenting with different ingredients and flavors can keep snack time exciting and enjoyable.

Overall, quick and easy snacks play a valuable role in a balanced diet, providing convenient and nutritious options to fuel your body and keep you going strong throughout the day. Incorporating a variety of energy-boosting snack ideas and nutritious snacks for on-the-go can help you stay satisfied, energized, and focused on your daily activities.

CHAPTER 9
Desserts For Treat And Nutrition

When it comes to desserts that offer both a treat for the taste buds and nutritional benefits, there's a wide array of options to explore. Healthy dessert choices have become increasingly popular as people look for ways to satisfy their sweet cravings without compromising their health goals. These desserts often incorporate nutrient-dense ingredients, natural sweeteners, and creative combinations that deliver both flavor and nourishment.

One category of healthy desserts focuses on incorporating fruits, nuts, and whole grains. Fruit-based desserts, such as berry parfaits, mango sorbet, or apple cinnamon crumble, are not only delicious but also packed with vitamins, antioxidants, and fiber. Nuts and seeds can add a crunchy texture and healthy fats to desserts like almond and date energy balls or chia seed pudding. Whole grains like oats and quinoa can be used to create hearty yet nutritious treats like baked oatmeal squares or quinoa chocolate chip cookies.

Another aspect of healthy dessert options is the use of alternative sweeteners. Instead of refined sugars, recipes may use natural sweeteners like honey, maple syrup, or dates. These sweeteners not only add sweetness but also bring additional nutrients and flavors to the dessert.

For example, a dessert sweetened with honey may have added antibacterial properties, while dates offer fiber and minerals along with sweetness.

Incorporating superfoods into desserts is also a trend in healthy dessert options. Superfoods like cacao, matcha, acai, and spirulina not only enhance the flavor but also contribute antioxidants, vitamins, and minerals. For instance, a chocolate avocado mousse made with cacao powder and avocado provides a rich, creamy texture along with heart-healthy fats and antioxidants.

Furthermore, the concept of healthy desserts extends to catering to specific dietary preferences and restrictions. There are numerous dessert recipes tailored for vegan, gluten-free, paleo, and keto diets. These desserts use alternative ingredients like coconut flour, almond flour, or plant-based milk to accommodate various dietary needs without compromising taste or texture. Examples include vegan chocolate avocado brownies, gluten-free almond flour cake, or keto-friendly cheesecake made with almond crust and stevia.

On the other end of the spectrum, indulgent treats with nutritional benefits offer a different approach to dessert enjoyment. These treats focus on using high-quality ingredients in moderation to create decadent desserts that still provide some nutritional value. For example, a dark chocolate mousse made with high cocoa content chocolate offers antioxidants and flavonoids while satisfying chocolate cravings. Similarly, a small portion of artisanal ice cream made with real fruits and organic dairy can be a delightful treat without excessive sugars or additives.

Nutrient-dense ingredients like Greek yogurt, coconut cream, and avocado are often used in indulgent treats to create creamy textures and add nutritional value. For instance, a Greek yogurt parfait with layers of fresh fruits and nuts provides protein, probiotics, and healthy fats alongside sweetness. Avocado chocolate truffles or coconut cream-based desserts offer richness and creaminess without relying heavily on traditional dairy or sugar-laden ingredients.

Moreover, incorporating herbs and spices into indulgent treats can elevate both flavor and health benefits. Cinnamon, ginger, turmeric, and cardamom not only add depth to desserts but also have anti-inflammatory and antioxidant properties. Desserts like chai-spiced cookies, turmeric golden milk ice cream, or ginger-infused panna cotta showcase how these ingredients can transform indulgent treats into health-supportive delights.

desserts that combine treat and nutrition encompass a diverse range of options catering to various dietary preferences, ingredient choices, and health goals. From fruit-based delights to indulgent treats with nutrient-rich ingredients, these desserts offer a delicious way to enjoy sweets while nourishing the body with essential nutrients, antioxidants, and wholesome flavors.

CHAPTER 10
Meal Plans For Ovarian Cancer Recovery

When designing meal plans for ovarian cancer recovery, several key concepts come into play to ensure they are effective and tailored to individual needs. Weekly meal plans should be comprehensive, balancing nutrition, taste, and ease of preparation. Additionally, meal prep strategies can significantly enhance convenience and adherence to the plan. Customizing meal plans for individual patients considers their specific dietary needs, preferences, and any treatment-related challenges they may face.

Weekly meal plans for ovarian cancer recovery should focus on providing a variety of nutrient-dense foods to support overall health and well-being. This includes incorporating a range of fruits, vegetables, whole grains, lean proteins, and healthy fats. The meals should be balanced in macronutrients (carbohydrates, proteins, and fats) and micronutrients (vitamins and minerals) to support immune function, energy levels, and overall recovery.

In designing meal plans, it's crucial to consider different dietary needs that patients with ovarian cancer may have. For example, some patients may have dietary restrictions due to treatment side effects such as nausea, taste changes, or digestive issues. Others may follow specific diets like vegetarian, gluten-free, or low-sodium diets. Tailoring meal plans to accommodate these needs ensures that patients can adhere to the plan and obtain the necessary nutrients for recovery.

Meal prep strategies play a vital role in the success of meal plans for ovarian cancer recovery. Preparing meals in advance can save time and energy, making it easier for patients to follow their dietary guidelines. This may involve batch cooking, where multiple servings of meals are prepared and stored for later use. It can also include pre-cutting vegetables, marinating proteins, or assembling ingredients for quick and easy meals during busy days.

Customizing meal plans for individual patients takes into account their unique circumstances and preferences. This may involve collaborating with a registered dietitian or nutritionist to assess nutritional needs, food preferences, and any challenges related to eating during treatment.

 For example, some patients may require higher calorie or protein intake to support weight maintenance or regain strength post-surgery. Others may benefit from specific foods or supplements to manage side effects like constipation or fatigue.

Incorporating variety and flexibility into meal plans is essential to prevent boredom and ensure a well-rounded diet. This includes trying new recipes, experimenting with different cooking methods, and incorporating seasonal produce for freshness and flavor. Additionally, encouraging patients to listen to their bodies and adjust portion sizes or food choices based on hunger cues and energy levels promotes a healthy relationship with food during recovery.

Overall, meal plans for ovarian cancer recovery should be holistic, taking into account nutritional needs, dietary preferences, meal prep strategies, and individualized support. By focusing on nutrient-dense foods, convenience, and customization, these meal plans can support patients in their journey towards healing and improved quality of life.

Conclusion

This guide delves into the crucial intersection of nutrition and oral cancer recovery. We begin by understanding the nuances of oral cancer and its relationship with nutrition. Highlighting key nutrients and dietary considerations, we explore foods that aid in recovery while steering clear of those that may hinder progress.

Moving into specific meal categories, we offer a comprehensive range of options tailored for oral cancer patients. Energizing breakfasts, wholesome main dishes rich in lean proteins and healing elements, brain-boosting salads, nourishing soups, memory-enhancing sandwiches, and snacks designed for quick energy are all included. We also delve into hydration strategies and brain-enhancing beverage recipes to support recovery.

Special occasion meals are not forgotten, with festive recipes that accommodate dietary restrictions. Lastly, we discuss effective meal planning and preparation strategies, offering customizable meal plans to meet varying needs. This holistic approach aims to empower patients with practical, nutritious choices throughout their oral cancer recovery journey.